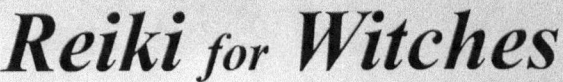

Reiki for Witches

A Multi-Purpose Holistic Tool for Witches, Wizards, Pagans and New-Agers

I0439859

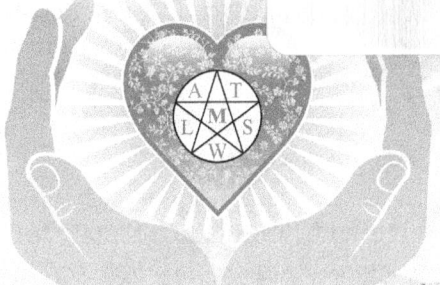

Dr. Isis Day

An Isis Day™ Publication

Books & Music By The Author:
For more information about these works, visit:
www.IsisDay.com

Books:

- JOAN OF ARC: A ROLE MODEL FOR WITCHES, WIZARDS, PAGANS AND NEW-AGERS : *How To Spiritually Achieve Whatever Your Mind Can Conceive.*

- REIKI FOR WITCHES : *A Multi-Purpose Holistic Tool For Witches, Wizards, Pagans and New-Agers.*

- WITCHES UNITE*! : Magic and Witchcraft : Our Gift, Our Heritage, Our Power!*

- MAGIC IS GOD; BLESSED BE! : *More Power to Witches, Wizards, Pagans and Witchcraft.*

- I AM A WITCH; I CHOOSE PAGANISM : *The Real Truth About Witches, Pagans, Magic and Witchcraft.*

Music CD Album:

- FULL MOON

About the Author:
Dr. Isis Day is a Witch, (thus, a Pagan). She's also a Spiritual/Holistic Practitioner, a Reiki Level III Master, a Vegan, a Spiritual Counselor, a Chaplain, a Certified Hypnotherapist and a Musician, with a doctorate degree in Pastoral Counseling Psychology. She resides in Houston, Texas, USA; her website is *www.IsisDay.com.*

REIKI *for* WITCHES
A MULTI-PURPOSE HOLISTIC TOOL FOR WITCHES, WIZARDS, PAGANS AND NEW-AGERS

By

Dr. Isis Day

Edited, Designed & Formatted by: Marie Guillaumes

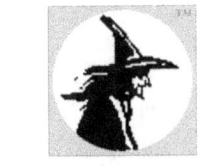

Isis Day™ Publishers
www.IsisDay.com

**REIKI for WITCHES:
A MULTI-PURPOSE HOLISTIC TOOL FOR
WITCHES, WIZARDS, PAGANS AND NEW-AGERS**

(*Black-&-White Interior Paperback Edition*)
First Edition — First Printing — Second Revision
Copyright © 2013, 2022 by Isis Day, Julius Williams,
Isis Day™ Publishers & JoDArc™ Publishers

Published by:
ISIS DAY™ PUBLISHERS
Houston, Texas, USA.
www.IsisDay.com

European Article Number (**EAN-13**):   **978-1482636437**
International Standard Book Number (**ISBN-13**):   **978-1-4826-3643-7**
International Standard Book Number (**ISBN-10**):   **1-4826-3643-3**

Isis Day™ Catalog Control Number (**ICCN**):   **IDID-1302-PB3A**

ACKNOWLEDGMENTS:

A very special thanks to my dear mom and grandma
— my highly beloved Mentors and Inspiration —
through whom I was born a Witch.

To my beloved brother, Osiris,
whose short life on earth triggered a curiosity
that awakened the Witch in me.

To Julius Williams and his loving family
whose friendship, support and influence I cherish very dearly.

I am very grateful to Magic — the Infinite Intelligence — for
Universal Life Force/Energy, and for EVERYTHING.

DEDICATED TO:

All Witches, Wizards, Pagans, New-Agers,
All Metaphysicians,
All Holistic Practitioners,
My Family, Friends, Relatives, Teachers & Mentors, and
All my Fans worldwide!

Reiki for Witches © 2013, 2022 Dr. Isis Day

TABLE OF CONTENTS

LIST OF FIGURES

FOREWORD:

We — Witches, Wizards, Pagans and New-Agers — are healers and thus naturally drawn to the healing Arts and Sciences, whether conventional or alternative. I consider Reiki a gentle unobtrusive part, expression or practice of Magic safely used in a new world where the old Pagan ways are frowned at and the practice of Witchcraft could attract dangerous and life-threatening antagonism if unwittingly done openly. Thus, as a part, Reiki cannot be greater than the whole — Magic. *Nothing can be greater than Magic.* Reiki cannot, therefore, replace Magic, as indeed nothing can. But Reiki brings or rather reveals something new to our practice, a new perspective that gives our Spells and Rituals an extra punch or momentum that promises faster, better and more lasting results. Sometimes in casting Spells or performing our Pagan rituals, we tend to focus or try so hard that it not only takes away the joy of practicing the Craft, but hinders success and progress, while putting a considerable strain and stress on us both emotionally and physically. Reiki teaches us that we are only supposed to 'Be There,' to be present, to simply let ourselves be the channel for the Universal Life Energy (Magic) to flow through and do its job. As a result, according to Reiki practice, we are to assume a simple relaxed approach and attitude toward the goal we seek to accomplish. This understanding gradually begins to shed a new exhilarating light on all we've known and all we do. Our Craft comes alive again renewing our joy of Magic, our love of who we truly are, and our desire to be even more of who we are and practice cheerfully. We are thus born again in a true sense of the words; all things are new; Magic is potent for us once more and not a drudgery; and life is not such a drag anymore. As a Witch, Wizard, contemporary Pagan or New-Ager, Reiki is like taking the remote control of your life with you wherever you go without fear of drawing negative attention to yourself and your Craft or practice. For times when you're away from your Temple or little private and sacred corner or even your Coven, group members or family, Reiki becomes a worthy companion that helps you stay in touch spiritually and do as much as is possible to remain holistically whole in every conceivable aspect of life — emotionally, physically, materially, socially, relationship-wise, career-wise, etc.

This book, 'REIKI FOR WITCHES: A MULTI-PURPOSE HOLISTIC TOOL FOR WITCHES, WIZARDS, PAGANS AND NEW-AGERS' is adapted from '*REIKI: A MULTI-PURPOSE HOLISTIC TOOL FOR METAPHYSICIANS,*' by Julius Miracle Williams, Ph.D.; (JoDArc Publishers). It was originally written as a school thesis and later modified for publication. You may read the details of the credits and modification in the Foreword of Mr. Williams' version of the book. If you've already read his, you don't really need to read mine.

I, Isis Day, so admire Mr. Williams' in-depth research and his simplified, humble, honest, lively and to-the-point style of writing that in addition to this book, I also opted to adapt another book of his – 'JOAN OF ARC: A ROLE MODEL FOR METAPHYSICIANS – *How To Spiritually Achieve Whatever Your Mind Can Conceive*;' (JoDArc Publishers). My version is entitled 'JOAN OF ARC: A ROLE MODEL FOR WITCHES, WIZARDS, PAGANS AND NEW-AGERS – *How To Spiritually Achieve Whatever Your Mind Can Conceive*;' (Isis Day Publishers). Check it out, and my other books too, including 'WITCHES UNITE*!*' and 'MAGIC IS GOD'; I'm sure you'd love them.

The significance of the letters in and around the pentagram on the cover of this book is explained in detail in my other book — 'WITCHES UNITE*!*' Basically, they are reminders (not quite a sigil); I combine them variously to say things like: 'Always Think Magic'

(ATM); See Magic Always (SMA); 'Magic Works' (MW); 'Live/Love Magic' (LM); the 'W' is also for Witch, Wizard and Witchcraft. I have the letters written all over, wherever I can (without the pentagram) — on my desk, in my car, on the mirror, mouse pad, etc.

It is my deepest wish that this book helps you become a better Holistic Practitioner — Witch, Wizard, Pagan or New-Ager — beyond your wildest dreams.

Like Julius Williams, I also believe in Love. Love heals! Love is the answer. With Love, all pains go away; and with lots of Love in our hearts, any good can be accomplished. Give Love a chance. Let Love reign in our hearts and everywhere. Love is Life. Love is all there is. The heart that loves lives, glows and grows. Let us therefore, Think Love, Act Love, Live Love, and Become Love! Thus, Love-A-Love-A-Day!! Reach Out And Love, universally and unconditionally!!!

Thanks for taking the time to read my book. May the best and most fun-filled experiences be your trademark, to the highest good of all concerned!

Don't forget to recommend this book positively to anyone you think could benefit from it. Do stay in touch. My contact information is on my website: www.IsisDay.com; Enjoy!
Namaste!!

— *Dr. Isis Day*
(*Houston, Texas, USA.*)
April 2013.

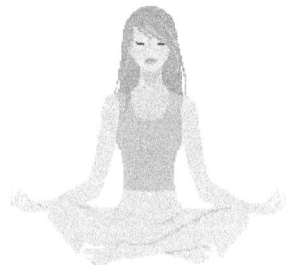

Blessed Be!!!

INTRODUCTION — CHAPTER 1

Reiki (pronounced *Ray-Key*), translates from the Japanese into 'Universal Life Force,' 'Universal Energy,' 'Vital Life Force,' 'Transfer of Energy' or "Universally Guided Energy" (Fernandez; 2003:6). Reiki, as a healing art, is fast becoming one of today's most popular emerging holistic practices, because of its ease of use, and the growing respect, success, and validity it has been achieving in recent years. This expository thesis discusses Reiki as an alternative type of healing practice, and looks at its significance within the context of Witchcraft, Pagan and New Age practices. It presents the history, concept and philosophy of this alternative therapy, which re-originated in Japan, but has existed for thousands of years, while focusing on its practice modalities, and why I consider it 'A Multi-Purpose Holistic Tool for Witches, Wizards, Pagans and New-Agers.' This paper also looks at the art and science of Reiki, and examines the key techniques associated with this Energy healing process which allows Practitioners to help themselves and others, thus healing the Inner Person through the use of this Universal Life Force (Magic) which "is found everywhere and in all things..." (Penczak; 2005:2)

While Reiki is not associated with any particular ideology, philosophy, religion, movement or organization, there are five main Principles and three major Degrees/Levels of Reiki Attunement and related Symbols passed down through the ages, which help to define Reiki methodology as a whole, and which are discussed in this paper. By applying these principles, it is believed that one is able to further enhance their own energy, providing a more balanced and pure life experience or Personal Transformation for themselves and others.

In this thesis, I also contend and explain why Reiki is not as complicated as some may erroneously think, and go further to discuss

Reiki as a holistic practice, and its usefulness in dealing with everyday issues like weight-loss, self-confidence, finances, stress, rejuvenation, relationships, aches, pains, and various other ailments. Reiki is an ancient ritualized laying-on of hands and a distant healing practice. It is the ability to heal through the Universal Life Force, wherever and whenever, by way of an Energy Healer acting as a channel for this Life Force. Reiki Practitioners believe that, "as well as being composed of energy... we also have energy running through us." (Parkes; 1998:15) In addition to cultivating discipline and responsibility, Pagans and New-Agers interested in exploring Reiki would be fascinated by Reiki's emphasis on, and use in, Chakra Balancing, because "Reiki healing operates through interaction between the Chakras and the endocrine glands." (Honervogt; 2008:37)

This paper shows how almost anything that makes humanity better in any way, could be easily and rightly dragged and dropped into the amazing world of Reiki, as "Reiki always works for the greatest good." (Vennells; 2000:64) The paper contributes to the Pagan Practitioner's knowledge and practice by drawing attention to the Multi-Purpose Holistic potential of Reiki, as well as by expanding and supporting previous information on Reiki. It describes the essence of Reiki, thus enabling Witches, Wizards, Pagans and New-Agers to better understand and practice this healing art as effortlessly as possible.

Finally, I will show my Reiki lineage right from the Reiki re-discoverer in our present time (within the last 200 years or so), Mr. Mikao Usui, down through my Honorable Reiki Master and Teacher, Julius Williams, and up to me. In the next chapter, I'll extensively review some of the books researched for this project as proof that there are tons of materials out there to help Practitioners get acquainted and involved with Reiki — a truly simple, flexible, beautiful and gracious art and science of Energy Healing, very suitable for Witches, Wizards, Pagans and New-Agers.

REVIEW OF LITERATURE — CHAPTER 2

"Reiki is a catalyst for growth and positivity in all areas of life..."
— Carmen Fernandez (2003:90) —

When I first got curious about Reiki nearly six years ago, **'Step-by-Step Reiki: How To Channel The Power of Natural Healing Energies'** by Carmen Fernandez (2003) was the first book I picked up. I had only read up to the third paragraph of the introductory page when I came across this line: "All you need is the desire to heal and be healed." (2003:6). It was astonishing, especially since it was my first step into the wonder-world of holistics. Further on, she writes: "Reiki embraces and enriches you and the people around you... You need no intellectual skills to use Reiki or to receive it." (2003:11) Fernandez then talked about how, following a Reiki attunement, "the ability to channel the power of Reiki is instant and everlasting." (2003:11) She holds that "Reiki is unconditional love in a world often beset by conflict, and it begins with you." (2003:11) I was sold! That was all I needed to hear to embrace Reiki; and the inspiration I've gotten from Reiki over the years is what has led me to research further and do this thesis on it.

News Flash! Magick meets Reiki!! Practitioners with a strong interest or background in Magick will be highly intrigued by Christopher Penczak's **'Magick of Reiki: Focused Energy for Healing, Ritual & Spiritual Development.'** (2005) In this groundbreaking examination of Reiki from a magickal perspective, Penczak adds new dimensions to the practice of Reiki, including 'New Age add-ons' such as 'Reiki Spirits,' and dives into the intersection of Reiki and Magick, and how these two amazing practices can be brought together with inter-connective possibilities. He gives an update on what else is going on in the field of Reiki, including how modern Magick Practitioners use Reiki Energy in their spells and rituals, what new facets are being included to the age-old healing art of Reiki, what other teachers and students are learning, and covers grounds that otherwise you would need to extensively research yourself. Penczak includes all the caveats, and all the potentials for using Reiki, and also suggests ways to integrate Reiki and magickal practice, such as using Reiki Energy for psychic development, using a Reiki Protection Shield, Reiki in Ritual and Spell work, Candle Magick, Crystals, Herbs, Flower Essences, Charms, Stones, Scents, Talismans, and much more. This is not a traditional Reiki book; and although you'll find much of the basic information about what Reiki is as a healing art, you won't find a conservative view of the art of Reiki. Penczak's personal experiences with other traditions serve as an open door for the reader to explore Reiki on a whole new level. The book is not just for those on a magickal path, but for those who are curious about Reiki and travel any spiritual path, with the willingness and courage to explore new frontiers in Metaphysics, or simply to broaden knowledge, and who would wish to turn their healing practice into a full-blown spiritual ascension system.

Penczak (2005) neatly shows that the basics of Reiki cannot be changed, for it is a Universal Energy, and when used for the higher good, is a very useful companion therapy. His writing style makes the topic very accessible and clear, is able to explore many views in a sensitive manner, is grounded in tradition, accessible in language, and creative in approach. In his book, he truly drives home my proposition in this thesis, that 'Reiki is a *worthy* Multi-Purpose

Holistic Tool for Witches, Wizards, Pagans and New-Agers,' especially since "Medical Reiki and Mystical Reiki are emerging as the two strongest schools of thought in the healing community today." (2005:4)

    Christopher Penczak (2005) is an Eclectic Witch, Writer, Healer, and a very gifted Teacher. His practice draws upon the foundation of modern Witchcraft, blended with the wisdom of mystical traditions from across the globe. Formerly based in the music industry, Penczak was empowered by his spiritual experiences to live a magickal life, and began a full-time practice of teaching, writing, and seeing clients. His book, 'Magick of Reiki' was the 2005 Coalition of Visionary Resources (COVR) Winner for Best Alternative Health Book!

    One of my favorite books on Reiki is '**Sacred Path of REIKI: Healing As A Spiritual Discipline**,' by Katalin Koda (2008). Two of the many things I've learned so far from my metaphysical and Pagan lessons is to try and 'turn adversities into blessings,' and also to 'keep all channels open' for blessings. Koda's book echoes these two concepts from an intriguing personal experience and accomplishment. When she was only nineteen years old, she learned to her dismay that she had Hodgkin's disease — a treatable cancer that grows in the lymph system. After six months of chemotherapy and being exposed to every kind of needle and blood worker in the clinic, she emerged healed, curious, and revitalized by her survival. Gradually, following her curiosity, it began to dawn on her that her cancer journey was truly a 'spiritual transformation,' and that somehow, it wasn't just the chemotherapy that had cured her. She became fascinated with any New Age information she could lay hands on, and a series of synchronistic events followed, culminating in the uniqueness of her 'Reiki Warrior' approach to the teaching of Reiki, which combines traditional Reiki techniques with Chakra healing, Hatha and Kundalini Yoga, Vegan/Vegetarianism, the Tibetan Dharma, ancient Vedic knowledge from India, the magical and crafting arts and practical applications of Wicca, and her own spiritual and clairvoyant experience. Koda presents tested theories and original practices that demonstrate how to develop Reiki into an integrated healing system and transcendent spiritual path.

Katalin Koda is indeed a practicing Metaphysician, and her curriculum vitae is not only impressive, but inspiringly all-embracing in what I call her unconscious quest to use 'all open channels' in her holistic practice to heal herself and others in all aspects of life. She has been practicing and teaching all degrees of Reiki for more than a decade, and is a certified Sivananda Yoga instructor, providing Chakra and Human Energy Field training. She helped fuel my desire to write this thesis on Reiki as 'A Multi-Purpose Holistic Tool for Witches, Wizards, Pagans and New-Agers,' for this is exactly what she has ended up doing — integrating all she's learnt into one simple practice — Reiki. Koda writes: "... My years of Wiccan training, Meditation practice, Tibetan Buddhist studies, Yoga practice, and work with Shamanic Journeying all merged into an incredible fusion of various traditions in the wondrous and harmonious practice of Reiki healing... I have not given up any of my qualities of Wicca or Yoga or being a mother, but simply absorbed them into each other... I discover that awakening is within the practice of Reiki..." (2008:4)

Anyone who sincerely tries to know something about Reiki would most definitely get to hear about '**Hands of Light: A Guide to Healing Through the Human Energy Field**,' by Barbara

Brennan (1988). More than 60% of Reiki students, Practitioners, Teachers and books that I've come in contact with have talked about and recommended this book. No wonder it is the #2 best-seller in Holistic books on the Web. It has become a Reiki Classic and Essential Reference Book. My research for this thesis made me pay closer attention to the information in this book. To my surprise, it felt like I'd not read it before. The only explanation I have for this feeling is that my metaphysical and Pagan studies have raised my consciousness and opened my mind to comprehend deeper esoteric knowledge. Brennan says that "Many people want to take more responsibility now for their health. To make this change a smooth one, the best way is to integrate the methods that are available, so that healing can become very personal again, as it was at one time in our history." (1988:149) 'Integrate!' That's the word! And it's a call to Witches, Wizards, Pagans and New-Agers to 'integrate' Reiki into their existing practices. She encourages you to "... look deeper into yourself, and wider into the available alternative methods." (1988:253) Brennan wrote extensively on the Chakra and Aura from a scientific, transcendental and holistic perspective. A former NASA scientist and atmospheric physicist, Brennan provides the first in-depth study of the Human Energy Field, known as the 'Aura.' She's a Healer, Therapist, and Scientist who has devoted more than twenty years to the research and exploration of this Human Energy Field.

David Vennells is the winner of the 2000 Coalition of Visionary Resources (COVR) Award for best Alternative Health Book. In his awe-inspiring book, '**Reiki for Beginners: Mastering Natural Healing Techniques**' (2000), Vennells tells a challenging story of how, for four long years, he suffered with Post-Viral Syndrome after a serious disease. He was so weak he could not even hold his arms above his head to wash his hair. Over those years, he was also in a serious accident; spent his time in bed or being pushed around in a wheelchair, and suffered from clinical depression. One day, he went to a lecture and experienced a healing technique known as Reiki; and almost immediately, he started to feel better. Vennells then reveals the rest of his story, including how he was healed, how he learned Reiki and went ahead to become a Practitioner and teacher of this healing method. His book includes the history and techniques of this system in a clear and easy to understand manner. Vennells included many stories from people involved in Reiki, and talks about how you can use Reiki to heal yourself and others, even your pets, and how you can make Reiki a part of your daily life in order to bring more peace and creativity into your day-to-day activities. He teaches how to prepare for a Reiki Empowerment (initiation/attunement), and what to expect when you go through it, including how to place your hands on yourself or another when doing an attunement or healing, plus meditative techniques and other methods that can bring you peace, serenity and joy every day of your life, and how you can easily share that with others. Vennells really showed that you can use it to heal physical ailments, bring about relaxation, and improve your concentration and memory. He points out how Reiki can be used to complement and enhance other healing systems, and how Reiki can apply to you in many surprising situations. He certainly made it clear that "Reiki's natural healing intelligence works in complete harmony with other therapies, often without our noticing its subtle interventions." (2000:117)

      Reiki Outreach International — the world's leading organization for the promotion of Reiki healing, endorsed '**The Complete Reiki Tutor: A Structural Course to Achieve Professional Expertise**,' by Tanmaya Honervogt (2008). Her book is indeed a one-stop guide for Practitioners, Teachers and Students, providing an in-depth knowledge of Reiki, with accompanying step-by-step techniques and hand positions for the three Degrees. She goes further to provide a thorough foundation for self-healing, healing others, and distant healing. Included are Reiki treatments and support for relieving a wide range of common ailments and emotional issues, plus sound advice on preparing for Master training, setting up a professional Reiki practice, and handling therapist/client issues. One outstandingly fascinating thing about this book is that it is lavish with vivid photographs of real humans demonstrating the various hands-on positions and methods of Reiki practice.

      Honervogt's chapter on 'Using Reiki with Other Disciplines' is a heart-warming support for my proposal, that Reiki is indeed 'A Multi-Purpose Holistic Tool for Witches, Wizards, Pagans and New-Agers.' She says that "Reiki can be used in conjunction with a number of other healing therapies... It brings additional power to any form of healing-touch technique and flows automatically from healer to receiver." (2008:247) She goes further to provide a long list of existing therapies that have been known and verified to work effectively with Reiki, and how Practitioners in those areas "report that their work has positively changed and intensified since taking the First Degree." (2008:247) Tanmaya Honervogt is a Reiki

Master-Teacher, has been working with Reiki healing and Meditation since 1983, and regularly holds training sessions in Traditional Usui Reiki in Europe, Japan, Australia and the USA.

"As human beings, we all have a basic desire to contribute positively to the world and make a difference to fellow beings, as well as to improve and enjoy life as much as it is possible to do so." (Parkes; 1998:33) Chris and Penny Parkes are a typical example of how many Practitioners are drawn to holistic practices by a deep desire to help loved ones, as well as oneself, plus the general urge to heal the entire world of pain and sorrow. Watching their aging parents struggle with different ailments like cancer was so unbearable to the Parkes that they had to sieve through the maze of alternatives, including Quantum Mechanics/Physics, to see how they could pro-actively alleviate their parents' pains. All their findings seemed to point to one basic underlying principle, that *Everything Is Energy*." (1998:13) It became undoubtedly obvious to them that *there is a Life Force which flows through all living beings, whether animals, vegetables or minerals*. In their quest, they learned that Reiki refers to a technique which enables a person to become a channel for a far greater amount of this Universal Energy. They quickly went on to study Reiki and got their First Degree Initiation. The profound transformation resulting from this experience made the Parkes decide that Reiki would be their preoccupation for life. Chris Parkes finally trained as a Reiki Master, and established The Reiki School with his wife, Penny, to provide the highest quality Reiki training throughout Britain. The Parkes later put together a wealth of information on Reiki in a book entitled '**Reiki: The Essential Guide to the Ancient Healing Art**.' (1998)

Tantric Reiki is one of the best-kept and jealously guarded secrets among Reiki Masters. It is a unique method which unites lovers through the power of the all-embracing Reiki Energy, and increases the amount of love and the intensity of the sexual experience to a practically indescribable extent. '**Tantric Reiki: How to Use Reiki to Enhance Love and Sex**' by Gail Radford (2005), presents Reiki and its principles, and introduces everything that can be learned about Tantric sex, the erotic points in the body, the flow of sexual energy, and the reinforcement of Kundalini power. Radford goes ahead to point out that "The use of Reiki, together with Tantric sex teachings, magnifies and glorifies the energy connections, allowing total surrender, peace and ecstasy." (2005:7) She maintains that "When sex is truly spiritual, fulfilling and joyful, it can transform lives." (2005:48) I strongly agree! This echoes Dr. Leon Masters' advice on what I may call 'spiritual sex.' Most of the pencil graphics in this book are akin to those found in the 'Kama Sutra,' and might thus seem inappropriate to some readers; but these graphics, in addition to Radford's stubborn intent on revealing all the secrets that she could on Reiki, have earned her a fair dose of both criticisms and approvals.

Reiki is truly everywhere, as it could seamlessly be applicable and adaptable to any conceivable human experience. In my research to see how far one could stretch Reiki, I was stunned to see the amazing information Radford (2005) wanted to share with her audience. She is awesome. She is the co-author of 'The Complete Reiki Course,' (2001) which revealed Reiki to the world, and is a Reiki Master of the highest degree, sharing her knowledge via lectures worldwide.

Every book and Teacher that I've known on Reiki in particular, or Holistics in general, mentions the 'Chakras.' In practice, Reiki and the Chakra are inseparable twins, with the Chakra as a major component of the practice of Reiki; but in essence, they deal with the same Energy — the Universal Life Force — although terms used to reference them may vary greatly. Basically, to practice Reiki more effectively, a Practitioner needs a good understanding of the Chakras. So, I thought it worthwhile to pick up a book that is solely focused on the Chakras. '**A Handbook of Chakra Healing: Spiritual Practice for Health, Harmony, and Inner Peace**,' by Kalashatra Govinda (2002), is so comprehensive that one needs no other book on Chakras to get a grasp. Geared towards beginners as well as to more advanced students, Govinda's book teaches you what the Chakras are and how they function; and it offers effective programs for harmonizing the energy of the Chakras which will change your entire outlook on life, and thus "lead to marked improvements in physical and mental health, psychological stability, and inner peace." (2002:9) The book is simple, yet very informative, with great illustrations, tables, charts, and a clear presentation for people who have no previous knowledge of the Chakras.

Color Healing is an integral part of Chakra Healing. The same way that one hardly talks of Reiki without the Chakras, so is it near impossible to talk of the Chakras without the Colors associated with them. From a Reiki perspective, the distinction, however, is not usually obvious, as the two are seamlessly interwoven into the healing art and science of Reiki.

'The Complete Book of Color Healing: Practical Ways to Enhance Your Physical and Spiritual Well-Being,' by Lilian Verner-Bonds (2000), is the first book I picked up when I first got curious about Color Healing. I was highly intrigued and impressed by the simplicity and lavish graphics of this book. Indeed, color surrounds and affects everyone, but most of us take it for granted. Since "color and life are inseparable" (2000:6), Verner-Bonds encourages a greater awareness of color, and shows us how we can learn to appreciate, understand and use color on every level - physical, mental and emotional - to enhance well-being and improve life. "Color comes from light," she says, "and without light there is no life." (2000:6) Certain colors are life enhancing while others drain energy. Her book has practical information on ways to introduce color into different areas of daily life, in our dresses, foods, homes, work environments, healings, relationships, and how to use color for children. Lilian Verner-Bonds is a Color Expert, Psychic, Healer, International Lecturer, Teacher, Author, and one of the world's leading Clairvoyant Palmists. She lived in Finchley, London, at the time of her book's publication.

Enter the 'almighty' Meditation! Meditation indispensably joins Reiki and Chakra Healing to form a perfect triad. Meditation is a word that almost everybody hears all through life, but I could invariably say that only very few have a clue of what it's all about, or its importance in a truly, practical holistic life and practice. I never really understood the essence of Meditation until I read about it from my class lessons in Metaphysics and Paganism. The emphasis placed on Meditation in the lessons was as good as saying '*no Meditation, no Holistic Practice.*' So I decided to re-visit a beautiful book that I've had since my keen interest in Holistics — '**How to Meditate: Gain Focus and Serenity with Easy-to-Follow Techniques**,' by Doriel Hall (2005), which is also the last, but not the least, in my literature reviews.

With over 350 photographs and specially devised step-by-step sequences, Hall reveals techniques to help you live in the moment, love your life, and open yourself up freely to the people around you. Hall's (2005) book is highly recommended by a leading international Yoga and Reiki Master-Teacher and Zen Buddhist — Ken Simmons (Satya Prem). Hall states that "Meditation is both the means and the end..." (2005:6), and that "When Meditation becomes part of daily life, it can help us to improve the quality of all our interactions with the world around us." (2005:56)

'Meditation, Chakra and Reiki,' remind me of 'Faith, Hope and Charity.' Like Charity, Reiki (Universal Love/Life Energy), as an art and science, is awesome because with its virtually unrestricted and unlimited 'open-door' policy, it embodies, incorporates and accommodates every other holistic practice, concept and philosophy, including ways to transform daily mundane chores and routines into revitalizing physical, emotional and spiritual experiences. The books reviewed heretofore, are just a tiny glimpse into the amazing world of Reiki, in the hope that it would help Practitioners embrace Reiki as a true 'Multi-Purpose Holistic Tool For Witches, Wizards, Pagans and New-Agers.'

METHODS — CHAPTER 3

Reiki is probably the simplest form of healing and self-development system that exists! It is "non-denominational, and practiced by people of many different religions and cultures. You don't need to commit to a belief system in order to channel Reiki, or enjoy its benefits..." (Fernandez; 2003:6) The ability to practice Reiki cannot be learned in books. To practice Reiki, you need to receive an attunement from a Reiki Teacher/Master, which connects you to the Universal Source of Love, Light and Harmony. The attunement could be done in person or from a distance. Reiki is the Art of Channeling Life-Force Energy. It is an energy-healing system and not a manipulative system (hands moving the body). Reiki is distinct from Reflexology and Massage, but is sometimes confused with those and other hands-on healing arts.

A LITTLE HISTORY OF REIKI:

The practice of Reiki is said to have been around for about 3,000 years, with roots pointing to both Egypt and Tibet. Like most other ancient healing practices, it was lost, and remained so until the early part of the 20th century when it was re-discovered by a Japanese Buddhist Monk — Mikao Usui. (Because he was born in the 1800's, some indicate the 19th century for this re-discovery.) Usui taught "two thousand students, and trained sixteen teachers" (Koda; 2008:17) in this system, one of whom was his successor — Chujiro Hayashi, who later, in the 1930's, taught the system to Mrs. Hawayo Takata, a Hawaiian Japanese-American. Most of the Reiki practiced in the west come from the teachings of Mrs. Takata, who directly "trained twenty-two Masters between 1970 and 1980" (Koda; 2008:18), including her daughter — Mrs. Phyllis Furumoto.

MY REIKI LINEAGE:

Virtually every Reiki Practitioner is interested in their lineage, since the system is not learned, but passed on via attunements. This is also because Reiki Teachers and Masters hardly ever fail to draw the student's attention to his or her lineage, from the re-discoverer, Mikao Usui, up to the Teacher/Master. Nearly all the Masters in the west and the rest of the world spring from Mrs. Takata's original twenty-two Masters. My lineage therefore, as handed to me by my Honorable Reiki Teacher and Master is as follows:

> Mikao Usui
> Chujiro Hayashi
> Hawayo Takata
> Phyllis Furumoto
> Pat Jack
> Cherie Wine-Prasuhn
> Jo Long
> Julius Williams
> Isis Day

THE FIVE ETHICAL PRINCIPLES (AFFIRMATIONS) OF REIKI:

The practice of Reiki strongly adheres to its founding principles as the secret of inviting happiness through many blessings, and the spiritual medicine for all illness. It also enjoins its Practitioners to think the principles in their minds, chant them with their mouths, in the morning and at night, with hands held in prayer. They are the heart of Reiki. Although there are several forms of the principles, Penczak's (2005) teacher taught him the following:

> "JUST FOR TODAY, I WILL BE GRATEFUL;
> JUST FOR TODAY, I WILL NOT ANGER;

JUST FOR TODAY, I WILL NOT WORRY;
JUST FOR TODAY, I WILL DO MY WORK HONESTLY;
JUST FOR TODAY, I WILL RESPECT ALL LIFE." (2005:24)

Usui taught that dedication to the principles, and living them, was essential to bringing about compassion, enlightenment, peace, kindness toward all, calm in the mind, and in one's life.

THE THREE DEGREES OR LEVELS OF REIKI ATTUNEMENT OR INITIATION:

A Reiki Attunement (or Initiation) is a simple ceremony that enables the recipient to permanently open up to the Universal Life Force on all levels (mental, physical, emotional and psychic), and is performed by a Reiki Teacher/Master trained to pass on the attunements. It is a process whereby your ability to channel the Reiki Energy is activated, and "with each degree, you become a wider channel through which Reiki healing energy can flow." (Honervogt; 2008:52) The process also clears and balances many energy channels within the body. It is always a special spiritual experience for the receiver and the Master. Attunement is usually given during Reiki instruction classes. You cannot be attuned against your will. You could refuse to accept an attunement! However, "once you have been attuned, if your hands are placed on someone, including yourself, then your Reiki channel is 'on.'" (Penczak; 2005:36)

Reiki is mostly taught in three formal degrees/levels as instituted by the re-discoverer, although some Teachers have slightly modified the number and content to suit their healing philosophy.

Training and practice of each level enhances growth and mastery of Reiki. The three Levels are designated I, II and III, with III being the Master Level. In Level one, people are taught basic techniques for hands-on treatments for self and others. This 1st-level class starts your Reiki flow, and you find out about Reiki history. In Level two one learns techniques for remote/distant healing, and receives attunement for using symbols to activate specific functions for mental and emotional healing, and for increasing the connection and effect of Reiki. After this degree, you can become a Reiki Practitioner. Level three adds a spiritual or intuitive healing energy function, and the ability to teach and attune others to use Reiki themselves. Each level requires an attunement or set of attunements. As one progresses through the levels, there can be a distinct and noticeable difference in the perception of effects and sensations for both the Practitioner and the client.

The third-degree/level Reiki is frequently divided into two parts; the first focuses on the fourth Reiki symbol and Master-level techniques, while the second part, depending on the school, focuses on how to teach Reiki to, and attune, others. In some Reiki systems there is a distinction between the Master and Master-Teacher levels. To learn to attune others, one must undertake a further teacher level, but some teachers teach and transmit a unified Reiki attunement which includes all the functions of the three levels, including the teacher functions.

HOW REIKI WORKS:

How Reiki works is a mystery that no one knows. The re-discoverer himself, Mikao Usui, said he does not know how to explain it. It simply works! Fernandez (2003) writes: "The way is beyond language, for in it, there is no yesterday, no tomorrow, no today." (2003:32) However, according to Verner-Bonds (2000), "healing therapies such as Acupuncture, Acupressure, Reiki, and the laying-on of hands, are all built on the premise that the body's energy flows can be influenced in a positive way through outside intervention." (2000:94)

In Reiki, you do not use your own energy, but rather become a channel that lets the Universal Life Energy flow through you to the recipient. Thus, unlike some other healing practices, Reiki does not deplete the Practitioner's energy, and would heal without draining the Practitioner, as well as benefit both the Practitioner and the recipient. The goal is to *recognize the Universe as a vibrant energy field, where all parts contain a vibrating Life Energy*. The healer, then, simply channels the energy from the Life Force of the Universe, using it to restore the balance of energy in the client.

With Reiki, there is no over-dose; the body only absorbs the healing energy it needs. Reiki is self-grounding, and has built-in protections. Reiki heals on all levels, as the energy is directed to all major organs, glands, body joints and chakras. Simply put, Reiki Energy goes where the recipients body needs it most. Reiki knows no boundaries in terms of time and space, and thus, would heal effectively, whether the person is within your touch, or remotely miles away from you.

REIKI HAND POSITIONS:

Reiki is mostly administered by a gentle non-invasive laying-on of hands near, and sometimes on, an individual, with the intent to assist the body with its own natural healing ability. It helps bring us back into harmony with the Universal Life Energy, which increases the body's ability to heal physical ailments, thus speeding up the recovery process. The simplest treatment involves the placement of one of the healer's hands on the head of the client, while the other is placed on the upper back. Although the re-discoverer of Reiki, Mikao Usui, used and taught five hand positions, the number of hand positions has grown over the years to twelve or more; but the seven most common hand positions are relatively simple to do, and generally correspond to the positions of the seven basic Chakra points based on the ancient metaphysical notion that "the human body has seven 'energy centers.'" (Radford, 2005:32). The hand positions for treating others is the same as for treating self; (*see figures 1 to 6; pages 34 to 39*). Reiki does not use massage or tissue manipulation. Nothing in Reiki resembles Massage. Your hands are simply held gently on or over each position until the energy ebbs. A little bit of intention or attention is needed but not intense effort or will. Reiki touch is very light. No pressure is applied.

REIKI SYMBOLS:

Reiki Symbols are a distinctive and empowering feature of the Reiki system of healing. These symbols act as links to connect the student with the Reiki Energy for life. When you are initiated into the Reiki system, the symbols and Reiki Energy are transmitted together during the attunement process. Forever after, if you think of, draw out, or say the name of the symbol, the associated aspect of the Reiki Energy is called forth. In the past (even nowadays), some Reiki teachers and authors sought to keep the symbols secret as a way to protect their value and keep them 'pure.'   However, with the emergence of the Internet, many authors of books and websites continue to reveal the symbols to the public; (*see figures 7, 8 and 9; pages 40 to 42*).

SOME REIKI HAND POSITIONS FOR SELF-TREATMENT

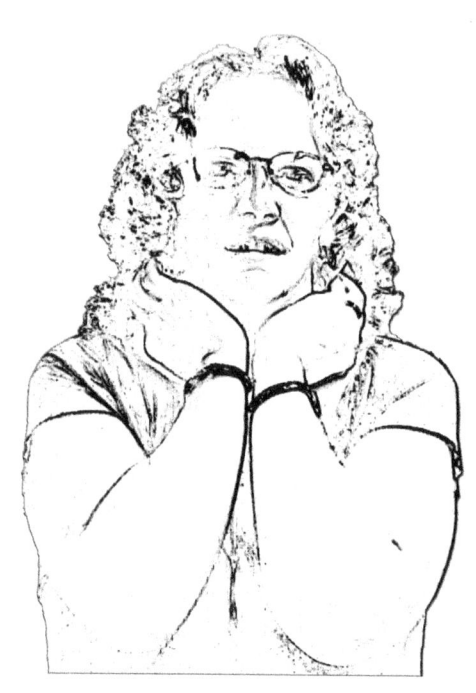

Figure 1

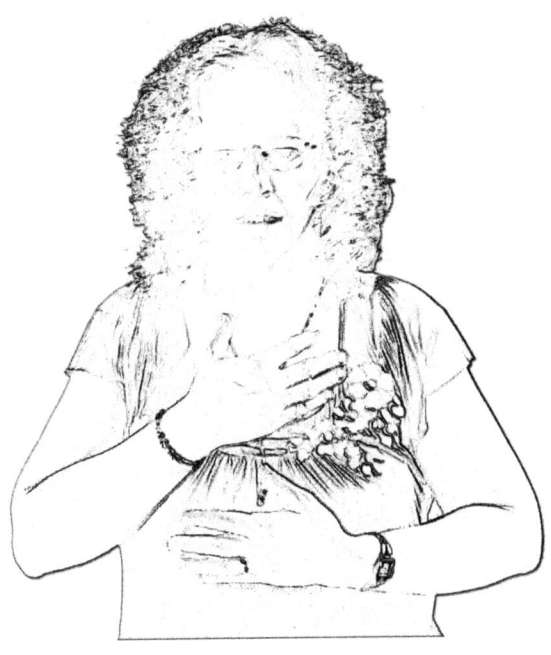

Figure 2

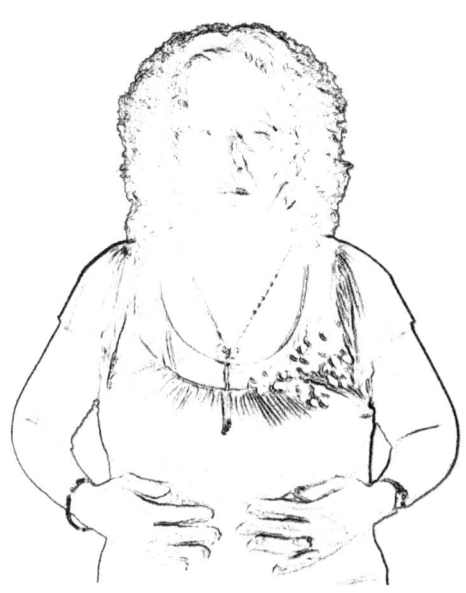

Figure 3

Some Reiki Hand Positions For Treating Others:

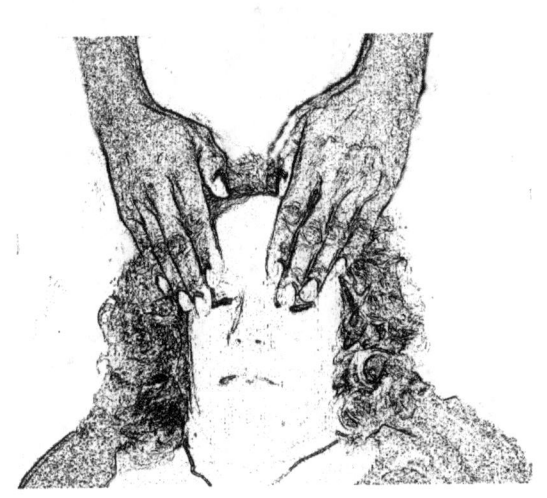

Figure 4

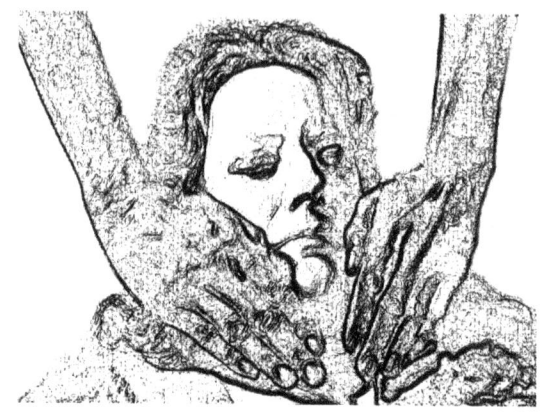

Figure 5

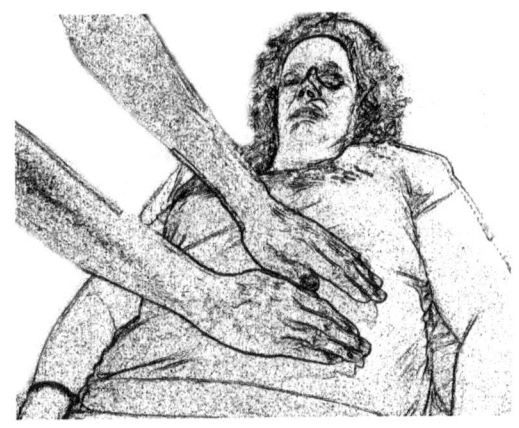

Figure 6

SOME REIKI SYMBOLS:

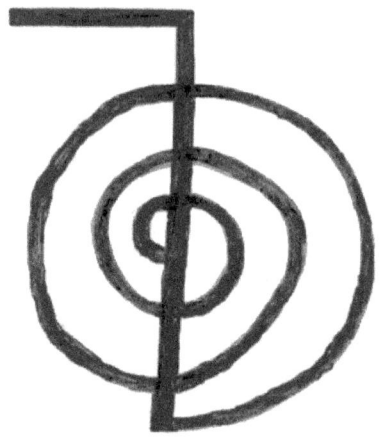

(Figure 7)

Cho-Ku-Rei
(*The Power Symbol*)

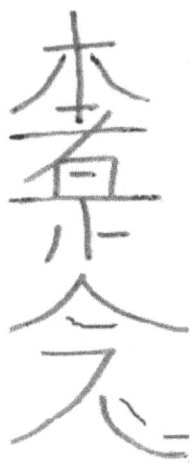

(Figure 8)

Hon-Sha-Ze-Sho-Nen
(*The Remote-Healing Symbol*)

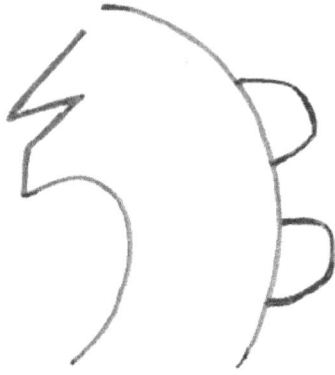

(Figure 9)

Sei-He-Ki
(*The Emotional Symbol*)

FINDINGS — CHAPTER 4

Reiki is a Holistic gumbo, a very flexible healing practice that incorporates an inexhaustible number of holistic, natural, alternative and complementary healing therapies, which makes Reiki very suitable for the versatile Practitioner. It is an excellent all-purpose system, easy to learn, and is not burdened with a lot of esotericism or dogma. It harmonizes well with most spiritual belief systems that allow for the existence of energy work.

The mystery of Reiki also stretches beyond mental, emotional, spiritual and physiological treatments and healings for humans, because it is equally very much used for animal and plant treatments, as well as for in-animate property blessings and treatments, including abstracts like prosperity, success and career treatments, or even for everyday basic necessities like clearing traffic and finding a parking space. Reiki can be used to manifest whatever you want. Reiki is versatile. Vennells (2000) says he would like to use Reiki in everything he does, to improve his quality of life, help his family, friends, and everyone he meets. He goes further to admonish that "We don't have to limit our intentions; we can have as many as we wish, or just one. We can set intentions for minor things... or for more important things... On a greater scale, we can use Reiki for healing conflicts or disaster locally, nationally, or globally." (2000:61) In fact, "You can bless all things with Reiki hands, including your food and drink." (Fernandez; 2003:34) And, combining Reiki and the Tantra, "we can use our body and its energies to lift our existence beyond the limits of the five bodily senses and rise to a cosmic level. Time and space become non-existent as we achieve the ultimate experience." (Radford; 2005:47)

Since the Universal Life Force upon which the practice of

Reiki is based is omnipotent and omnipresent, Reiki is also considered equally omnipotent and omnipresent, which is why it is easily applicable and adaptable to all aspects of life involving human, animal and plant needs and welfare. Once attuned to practice Reiki, virtually anyone, from all walks of life, can administer this important healing art, which definitely transcends gender, race and age, and unifies us all into a Universal Energy Field of growth and wholeness. Respected Reiki Masters and Practitioners believe that everyone is born with Reiki, given that Reiki is an expression of the 'Universal Energy of Life' itself. It is practiced worldwide by various cultures and religions, including Christians, Buddhists, New Age and contemporary Pagans.

Meditation, the number one friend and tool of the Metaphysician, is also a key ingredient in the practice of Reiki, making it easy for Reiki to be adopted into regular holistic activities. Those who are interested in Yoga, Aroma Therapy, Reflexology, Chakra Healing, Chroma/Color Therapy, Feng Shui, Witchcraft and other Pagan rituals, will also find that Reiki could be an integral part of such practices. "Reiki is so inclusive in nature that it complements all other healing arts, especially tactile ones..." (Fernandez; 2003:86) But, "unlike many healing arts, Reiki can be administered anywhere, anytime, and under most conditions. The recipient... need not even be physically present." (Radford; 2005:28)

Reiki Energy works to harmonize, or bring into balance, the total you. It enhances the body's natural ability to heal itself. It increases vitality and stamina, works throughout the body, on the mind, emotions, spiritual essence and aura. Reiki treatment releases blocked energy, promotes relaxation and reduces stress. Reiki Energy has an innate intelligence and goes wherever needed in the body and aura. It helps to cleanse the body of toxins, both energetic and physical, and can, over time, enhance intuition, Meditation and spiritual evolution. In addition, it enhances other body works, healing techniques and sports performances, and even treats and energizes you while you are treating others.

Reiki also works on machines and appliances, and has been used for treatment of world events. The Reiki system is a simple and powerful system of energy work. When you use Reiki, you find many more ways to work with, and gain value from it. The possible ways and systems for working with Universal Energy are infinite.

The use of Reiki as a relaxation and stress reducing technique, in addition to its use in supporting treatment of illness and injury, is becoming accepted and widespread. Many people like to get regular hands-on Reiki treatments as a refreshing and relaxing treat for themselves, in the same way that they might get a Massage, a facial, a guided visualization session, or a mud bath. Reiki can be a door to a higher part of your own spiritual being.

Only a slight amount of attention is needed to keep Reiki flowing. It does not involve mental strain or intense will, just a subtle intention and willingness. You are not pushing the Reiki Energy, you are allowing it to flow through you like water flows through a hose. The basic Reiki Energy has always been intention activated. The most important thing is to use Reiki often. The more you use it, the more comfortable, confident and skilled you will become. Usually the Reiki Practitioner feels rested and revitalized after the treatment. You might experience normal tiredness from standing a long time if you are not used to doing so. Any unusual tiredness usually indicates that the Practitioner has been forcing the energy or pushing with personal will rather than *allowing* the Reiki Energy to flow naturally.

Science is reluctant to accept the validity of energy work but double-blind studies have often shown significant and accelerated improvement from energy treatments of many different forms. Kirlian and aura photographs have shown significant changes before and after Reiki treatments, and "have revealed that the nature of the 'unseen energy' that all living things possess can be positively influenced by the application of Reiki treatments." (Honervogt; 2008:18)

Sometimes people have unreasonable expectations of Reiki both as clients and as Practitioners. Reiki does not often confer an instant miraculous cure of any condition. Reiki works with you to restore energetic balance and repair things like blockages, tears and wears in the energy field which create disease and unhappiness, and this can sometimes take time. This is why the Practitioner is usually admonished not to focus on, and be attached to, outcomes, but to *simply allow the energy to flow as effortlessly as possible.*

Relaxation is probably one of the primary reasons people try Reiki. If you need to relax, Reiki is a healthier choice than using alcohol, drugs, sugar, or other substances. Reiki gives you a break from pain, enhances the healing effects, and reduces the side effects, of any conventional or alternative medications you are taking. It reduces the time you need to heal after surgery, promoting your body's own internal healing system. It helps you release stuck or buried emotions, giving you a pure sense of love, as Reiki Energy is the energy of love. Love contains the power of the Universe and brings forth a sense of wholeness and connection. "Reiki certainly nurtures imagination and creativity too." (Fernandez; 2003:19) If you're feeling stuck or looking for resolution of a specific issue, Reiki can help. While you're having a Reiki session, you may experience an Aha! moment; you may have a realization or insight that answers a question or solves a problem, or you may find that the solution comes to you in your dreams or unexpectedly in the next few days.

"Reiki has grown tremendously in popularity over the last ten years or so, and treatment is now widely available at nearly every holistic clinic or complementary medicine centre in Britain, Europe, the USA, Australia and many other countries." (Parkes; 1998:39) In some Chiropractors' offices, Clinics, Spas, Hospitals and other health care settings, Reiki is given as a formal treatment. Many traditional health care providers have learned Reiki and integrated it into their practice, and more are doing so all the time; and it has become evident that "Medical Doctors, Chiropractors, Homeopaths, Healers, Therapists, Acupuncturists, etc. will all work together to aid the healing process." (Brennan; 1988:151) Books like 'Reiki Energy Medicine' by medical social worker — Libby Barnett et al (1996), and 'Reiki and Medicine' by physician Nancy Eos (1995), which describe the authors' experiences using Reiki at Massachusetts General Hospital and in other home, hospital and hospice settings, have called attention to Reiki as a complementary method of patient care. In some states, nurses now take Reiki classes to fill continuing education course requirements.

PERMISSIONS:

Reiki is a non-intrusive process, and would therefore not override any person's free will. This is why you would need a person's permission to give them Reiki treatment or attunement. To treat a minor or pets and plants, you'd need the custodian's permission, if any. The general ethical rule is that you do not give/send treatment without permission; but if you intend that Reiki be offered, accepted, and sent to where it is needed most, it will usually be accepted by the person or being you're offering to treat, as long as you intend it 'for the highest good of all concerned.'

It is important to keep in mind that Reiki is as effective without touch as it is with touch. Although touch adds a beautiful and therapeutic element to the practice, and is a basic need for everyone, it is essential that Reiki Practitioners never insist upon the touch aspect of Reiki, or impose it on someone who does not feel ready or comfortable with it. A Reiki recipient may shy away from touch either because not everyone is psychologically capable of dealing with touch, or for whatever personal, religious, cultural, ethical or gender reasons. The Practitioner should therefore not hesitate to discuss this with a client before giving treatment. In fact, according to Penczak (2005), because of legal concerns regarding touch and body privacy issues, some Reiki Practitioners in certain areas practice Reiki without touch. They simply hold their hands over the body. Thus, "a new movement has grown in the Reiki world called 'hands-off.'" (2005:59)

CAUTION:

The practice of Reiki does not ignore or overlook existing legalities surrounding all practices in various fields, and a potential for malpractice claims exists. As an example, during a Reiki session, although you may place your hands on the receiver/client, you do not move/rub your hands on him/her, as that could be termed 'Massage,' and in most countries, you have to be certified to practice Massage or other therapies that allow for such. Ideally, a Reiki Practitioner respects the law and rules in his/her geographical area of practice, and seriously tries not to cross any lines, stated or implied.

Reiki is not a substitute for Medical treatment, nor is it a diagnostic system. As a Reiki Practitioner, you do not diagnose. We do not in any way attempt to locate or define medical (physiological or psychological) needs. You must take care not to alarm the client nor to violate laws against diagnosis by non-medical professionals. You may ask questions, make suggestions, or suggest they see a Doctor or Psychologist about areas of concern. The United States and many other countries have very severe penalties for practicing medicine without a license. Anyone seeking Reiki treatments who has a medical condition should be reminded to see an appropriate Practitioner.

Being a Reiki Master is not a sign or guarantee of a person's moral integrity, upstanding behavior, or any form of emotional or spiritual development. Reiki Practitioners are as human as anyone else, and standard precautions apply.

The subject of nudity and Reiki requires extreme caution.

There is never any reason to have anyone dis-robe in order to use Reiki. It is my opinion that Reiki sessions are to be conducted with both the giver and receiver fully, decently and comfortably clothed. If the energy can be sent distantly to heal, then it should have no problem passing through some simple fabric. I have heard that some schools teach that attunements have to be performed nude. This practice is never necessary and places the student in an awkward position that is grossly inappropriate. Nudity during Reiki sessions is a method that is not at all popular amongst serious Reiki Practitioners, and has long been frowned at by a great many students and Masters. The only exception upheld by such critics is if such nude treatments are given only by legit couples to each other, if they so please.

Finally, don't forget your client's golden need for 'Confidentiality,' 'Privacy,' 'Trust' and 'Respect.' Observe them diligently!

DISCUSSION — CHAPTER 5

"From the perspective of a healer,
illness is the result of imbalance.
Imbalance is a result of forgetting who you are.
Forgetting who you are creates thoughts and actions
that lead to an unhealthy lifestyle
and eventually to illness."
— Barbara Brennan (1988:131) —

Reiki can do no harm and cannot be used for any harmful purpose. Whether there is ultimately a cure or not, the goal of the practice of Reiki is to alleviate suffering and promote well-being. When we speak of healing, a well physical body may be the first thing that comes to mind. However, the root meaning of the word is 'whole.' The practice of healing is that of becoming whole on all levels of being — the physical, emotional, mental, and spiritual. Illness truly happens when the mind, body and spirit become unbalanced. When tensions develop in your physical body, or blocks occur in your mind or emotions, your flow of vital energy can stagnate and become depleted excessively. You start then to break down physically and emotionally, wondering if you will ever recover. You then begin to become separate from yourself, further alienating yourself from your source of Life Energy. This "separation promotes fear and victimhood; fear and victimhood only support the illusion of powerlessness." (Brennan; 1988: 133)

True health is reached only by returning the entire being to harmony and balance, not only with itself, but with the Earth and the Universe. *We begin healing by desiring to be well and whole.*

Without the motivation to be well, and the intention to act in our own behalf, we cannot become well. "Basically, any disease, disorder, or unhappiness is the result of some disharmony in the body, mind, or environment." (Vennells; 2000:155) Reiki helps us become whole in all ways; and "through Reiki, you can awaken a sense of wonder at the world around you and learn to appreciate all the simple pleasures that life has to offer everyday." (Honervogt; 2008:22)

Reiki relaxes, soothes and comforts. It relieves pain, reduces symptoms and accelerates healing. Reiki enlivens and nourishes every level of your being — physically, mentally, emotionally and spiritually. It is an effective technique for prevention of diseases and energy imbalances in your system, and is also a highly effective tool for personal transformation. The Reiki method of natural healing is designed to systematically strengthen your absorption of Vital Life Energy. When a person is already in good health, Reiki is good preventive medicine. When an individual is seriously or chronically ill, regular Reiki treatments can gradually restore the body's natural state of balance, normal function, and wellness, especially when used as a complement to conventional medicine. Even when someone is terminally ill, Reiki can ease suffering and enhance the quality of life.

"Reiki combines well with other complementary therapies, and indeed with conventional forms of medicine... Reiki combines well with Hypnotherapy." (Parkes; 1998:65) "Experience shows, however, that these different approaches work quite well together." (Govinda; 2002:13)

Because Reiki is timeless, limitless, and not restrained by space and boundaries, it can be applied to anything in existence made of energy, whether in the past, present, or future. The Parkes (1998) state that *"Physically we are all energy. Everything within and around us is made up of energy and we are all part of one great energy field."* (1998:14) Fernandez (2003) maintains that "Reiki is the energy of all life — guided by the wisdom of the Universe... Having its own intelligence, Reiki has no boundaries, yet it knows where it is most welcome..." (2003:10)

Koda (2008) reminds the Practitioner to keep in mind that "Reiki is not in any way a substitute for medical advice, counseling, or therapy," (2008:91), and that he/she should never diagnose or give counseling advice beyond his/her training. Reiki will however support and enhance any form of treatment. Reiki can be used to nourish and restore the body from everyday life stressors. Whether it is a ten minute or a full body session, this gentle Reiki Energy will allow the body to replenish and restore its natural immune system. Reiki can be used to aid the body's natural ability to heal headaches, exhaustion, colds, sleeplessness, injuries and any other form of 'dis-ease.' Reiki is available to everyone. Anyone of any age or illness level can receive Reiki. Even newborn babies or people at the end of life can benefit from the relaxation that Reiki provides. For the Practitioner, the key to all this "is simply integration and practice." (Koda; 2008:6)

SUMMARY AND CONCLUSIONS — CHAPTER 6

"Reiki can take us as far as we want to go
in whatever we wish to do."
— David Vennells (2000:61) —

With Reiki, you're never alone. As an expression of the 'Universal Life Force,' Reiki is truly everywhere. Reiki is all-inclusive. Reiki neatly and warmly embraces everything you've known and everything you'd ever know in terms of holistic practices, as it combines, includes, and gracefully integrates all metaphysical disciplines into one 'whole,' and thus '*w*holistically' complete. "Reiki can never be depleted." (Vennells; 2000:61)

For Practitioners, as more and more people continue to seek alternative solutions to the problems of the body, mind and spirit, Reiki has the potential of becoming an essential part of a Practitioner's daily and regular practice, since it offers many of the benefits of healing touch, without the drawbacks, thus helping Practitioners become skilled, compassionate and well balanced healers. "Those who practice Reflexology, Massage, Aromatherapy, Shiatsu, and other forms of bodywork find that their work is enhanced by combining it with Reiki." (Parkes; 1998:66)

The practice of Reiki does not require any credentials or licence. The only requirement is at least the Level 1 Attunement, and the sincere desire to help oneself and others. Since Reiki work uses Universal Energy, and since that energy is directed by will, the potential for Reiki is virtually limitless. Koda (2008) maintains that although Reiki can be used as a spiritual practice, "Reiki is not a religion," (2008:205), and does not promote any prescribed cultural activity. "Some do not call their practices spiritual at all." (Brennan; 1988:273) But, because Reiki is a universal method, the practice is open to all religions, including Christians, Buddhists, New Age and contemporary Pagans. It is impervious to racism, sexism, political or religious thoughts. Being attuned to Reiki does not entail any conversion or adoption of spiritual beliefs or practices from any religion or particular set of beliefs. Since the healing provided by a Reiki Practitioner is an impersonal process giving direct, unmediated access to the divine, it is available to anyone willing to learn the method.

As a healing energy, Reiki is considered to be positive (no harm can come from Reiki), and intelligent (the energy heals what is needed even if you don't consciously know what you need). The recipient draws the right amount of energy to exactly where it is needed. Reiki works to heal you at the root of any disease, imbalance, or disharmony.

Because Meditation is a popular practice of calm concentration that gradually eliminates the effects of external stimuli and produces a stress-free state and inner harmony, combining Reiki with Meditation greatly enhances the practice of Reiki, and vice versa; Reiki and Meditation successfully complement each other to help us "Abandon Unhappiness and Develop Happiness." (Vennells; 2000:140) "Whilst being attuned, participants in Reiki workshops find that they naturally slip into a meditative state, even if they have never meditated before." (Parkes; 1998:67)

Within the Pagan context, I say Reiki is Magic at work — an

expression or gentle practice of Magic. Reiki is the easiest and cheapest Healing Therapy anyone can practice. Unlike most other healing methods, Reiki requires no acquisition of tools or equipment, nothing to carry about with you; although you may choose to decorate your practice room (if any) to suit the mood, including some light music. Wherever you are, Reiki is there ready to work, for like Magic, it is everywhere — omnipresent.

Finally, Reiki is a technique for total healing, stress reduction and relaxation. Using Reiki Energy, it is possible to tap into the unlimited supply of the Universal Life Energy in order to improve health and enhance the quality of life. Potentials for Reiki strongly abound; and the best way to explore these potentials is to learn to use Reiki, or simply, just be Reiki! As Practitioners, "we must walk the talk and practice the Reiki that has been activated within. Only then can we begin to help heal those around us in our community and our world." (Koda; 2008:45) Brennan (1988) points out that "to become a healer means dedication. Not to any specific spiritual practice, religion, or set of rigid rules, but dedication to your particular path of truth and love... which... will probably change as you travel through your life." (1988:273) As with most things, practice makes perfect. Reiki is in the DOing and BEing! In giving Reiki, keep in mind that there is technically no wrong way to do it, and simply be free of expectations, while keeping the ego in check. Reiki will work, whether you and your client believe in it or not, and will therefore "simply facilitate holistic healing and promote well-being." (Fernandez; 2003:19) And that is one of the many qualities of Reiki that make it a truly 'Multi-Purpose Holistic Tool for Witches, Wizards, Pagans and New-Agers.'

"The spiritual journey is like a spiral path
up and around a mountain,
so that with each turn of the spiral,
you come back to the same point,
only higher up and with a wider view."
— Doriel Hall (2005:94) —

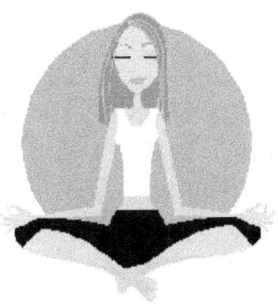

Blessed Be!!!

BIBLIOGRAPHY:

Brennan, Barbara 1988
 HANDS OF LIGHT: A GUIDE TO HEALING THROUGH THE
 HUMAN ENERGY FIELD.
 New York: Bantam Books.

Fernandez, Carmen 2003
 STEP-BY-STEP REIKI: HOW TO CHANNEL THE POWER OF
 NATURAL HEALING ENERGIES.
 London: Hermes House.

Govinda, Kalashatra 2002
 A HANDBOOK OF CHAKRA HEALING: SPIRITUAL PRACTICE
 FOR HEALTH, HARMONY, AND INNER PEACE.
 Old Saybrook, Connecticut: Konecky & Konecky.

Hall, Doriel 2005
 HOW TO MEDITATE: GAIN FOCUS AND SERENITY WITH
 EASY-TO-FOLLOW TECHNIQUES
 London: Hermes House.

Honervogt, Tanmaya 2008
 THE COMPLETE REIKI TUTOR: A STRUCTURAL COURSE TO
 ACHIEVE PROFESSIONAL EXPERTISE.
 London: Gaia.

Koda, Katalin 2008
SACRED PATH OF REIKI: HEALING AS A SPIRITUAL
DISCIPLINE.
Woodbury, Minnesota: Llewellyn Publications.

Parkes, Chris, and Penny Parkes 1998
REIKI: THE ESSENTIAL GUIDE TO THE ANCIENT HEALING
ART.
London: Vermilion.

Penczak, Christopher 2005
MAGICK OF REIKI: FOCUSED ENERGY FOR HEALING,
RITUAL & SPIRITUAL DEVELOPMENT.
St. Paul, Minnesota: Llewellyn Publications.

Radford, Gail 2005
TANTRIC REIKI: HOW TO USE REIKI TO ENHANCE LOVE AND
SEX.
Israel: Astrolog Publishing House.

Vennells, David 2000
REIKI FOR BEGINNERS: MASTERING NATURAL HEALING
TECHNIQUES.
St. Paul, Minnesota: Llewellyn Publications.

Verner-Bonds, Lilian 2000
THE COMPLETE BOOK OF COLOR HEALING: PRACTICAL WAYS TO ENHANCE YOUR PHYSICAL AND SPIRITUAL WELL-BEING.
New York: Sterling Publishing Company, Inc.

- - - - - - - - - - -

Day, Isis 2013
JOAN OF ARC: A ROLE MODEL FOR WITCHES, WIZARDS, PAGANS AND NEW-AGERS — *How To Spiritually Achieve Whatever Your Mind Can Conceive.*
Houston: Isis Day™ Publishers.

Day, Isis 2013
WITCHES UNITE! — *Magic and Witchcraft: Our Gift, Our Heritage, Our Power*!
Houston: Isis Day™ Publishers.

Day, Isis 2015
MAGIC IS GOD; BLESSED BE! — *More Power To Witches, Wizards, Pagans and Witchcraft.*
Houston: Isis Day™ Publishers.

Day, Isis 2021
I AM A WITCH; I CHOOSE PAGANISM — *The Real Truth About Witches, Pagans, Magic and Witchcraft.*
Houston: Isis Day™ Publishers.

Want more... ?

To place an order, or to find out more about our Books, Music, Movies, eBooks, Audio-Books, other publications and Free Downloads, contact or visit us at:

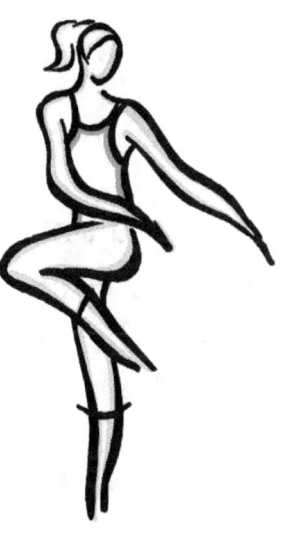

www.IsisDay.com

ISIS DAY™ PUBLISHERS

Houston, Texas, USA.

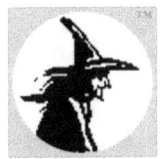

ISIS DAY™ PUBLISHERS
www.IsisDay.com

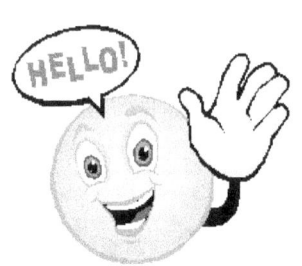
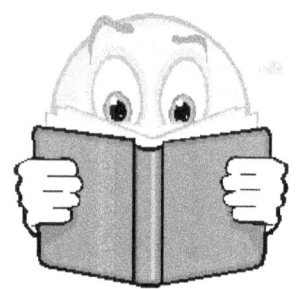

Have you optimistically told someone about this book lately? If not, kindly tell some folks right away, or give it to them as a gift.

And, do you have a link to it on your website(s) and email signature(s)? If not, here's the link to provide your audience:

WWW.ISISDAY.COM

Thank You !!!

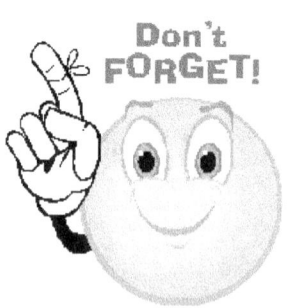

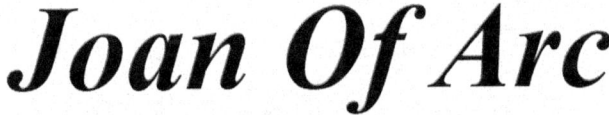

Joan Of Arc

A Role Model For Witches, Wizards, Pagans and New-Agers

How To Spiritually Achieve Whatever Your Mind Can Conceive

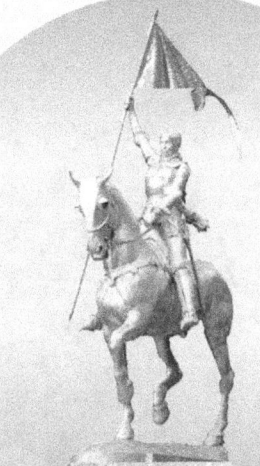

Dr. Isis Day

An Isis Day™ Publication

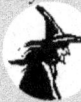

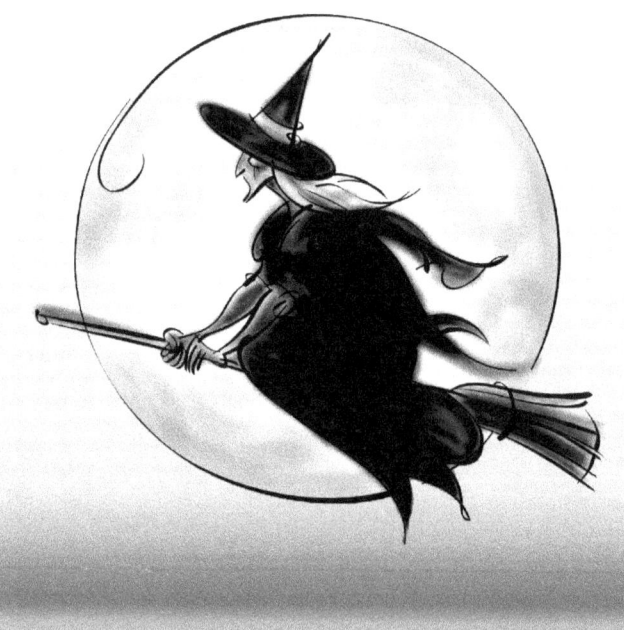

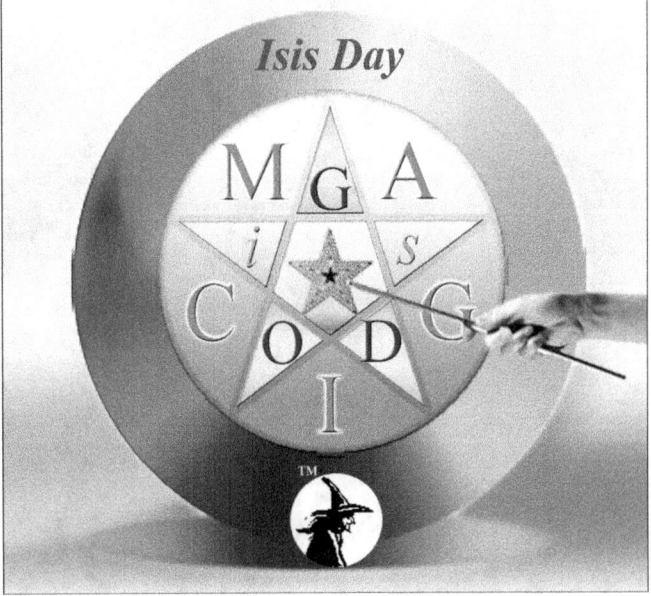

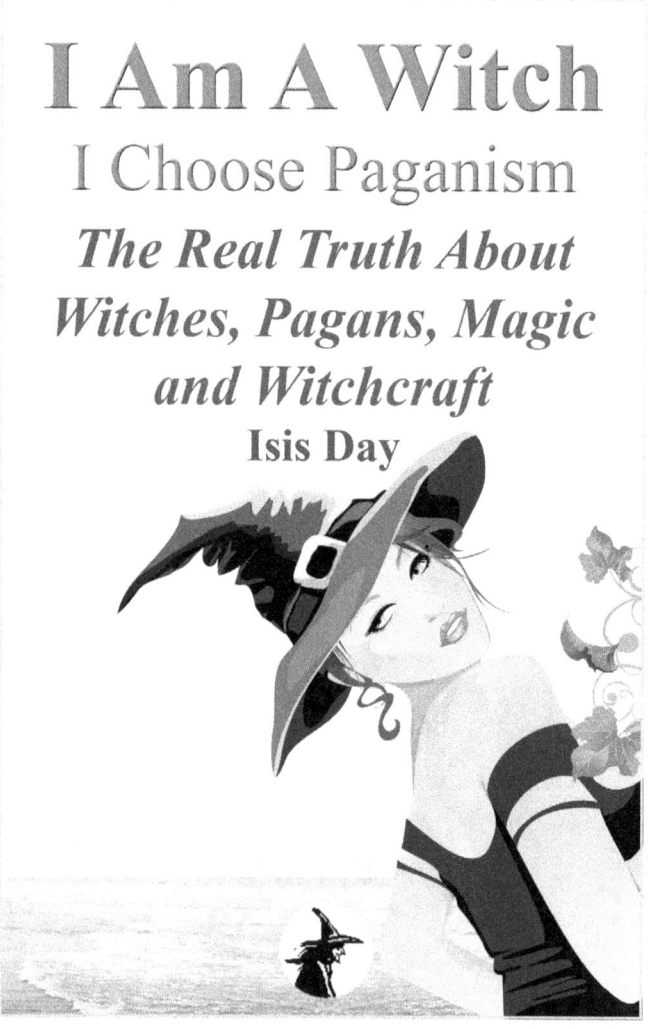

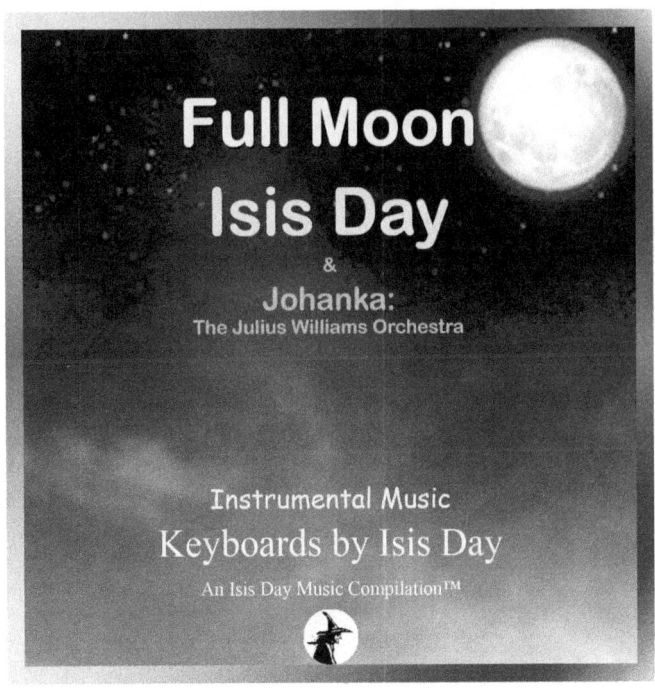

www.ingramcontent.com/pod-product-compliance
Lightning Source LLC
Chambersburg PA
CBHW070610290526
45790CB00002B/860